Canonizing the celebrity lifestyle and pop-culture is the condition unhappy people suffer from. Many dream of living in an enormous mansion, because Jay Z lives in one, or about the newest iPhone, since all celebrities seem to have it, the fast cars you see on TV, that seem to get the owners gorgeous blonde women, all of these things are showcased by social media and television as life-changing, as a gateway to the lifestyle of the successful, but what is success really? Is waking up in a gigantic mansion, with a partner that only makes you happy for your stuff and driving a sports car that only makes you happy because it turns the heads of people who don't even know your name success?

Or maybe success comes in some other form, and is found in a smaller apartment, shared with the person that makes you feel important? We, as humans, are constantly being fed with ads, commercials, depicting their product as one that comes with a designated lifestyle, while all they do is sell you dreams, dreams that vanish as fast as the joy those products bring you.

Forget about buying this, or buying that, forget about looking like one of those models who only eat once a day, or the guys with the pumped up muscles, forget about the need of having hundreds of phone numbers that you never touch, because all of that means nothing, when these items and expectations stop you from being happy, filling your mind with thoughts about what you don't have, instead of enjoying what you DO have.

Minimalism has one goal only, making YOU feel JOY, by eliminating the negativity in your life, in order to make room for happiness.

How it all began...

Unlike some other minimalism success stories, mine's a little different, I was not exactly unhappy, being born in a middle-class family I got all the necessities and some luxuries also, but the way I idolized some celebrities' lifestyle pushed me towards something I believed was right, something I imagined would bring me joy.

Soon enough, at the age of sixteen, my parents got me my first gym membership, and I loved it, later I got my first car, which was more than decent for an average kid, success with girls was not a problem, constant parties and nights spent in bars with plenty of friends, it looked like things were great, however, quite the contrary.

I would get up every morning sore from yesterday's workout, after having the same repetitive breakfast, my mind automatically drove me to the gym. After training, I had a coffee with one out of the same group of people, got home, ate all day long, in the evening whenever someone called to hang out my body would instinctively go, regardless of what I had to do the next day, and this kept repeating like a song put on replay, and I thought I was happy.

It all hit me during my first year of law school, when I woke up one morning sore as usual, and I refused going to the gym, something I never done before. And then it all came flashing down in my mind, I am spending all of this money, time and effort in the gym, just to maintain my six-pack so women will think I'm attractive, I constantly waste time and money in coffee shops and pubs since that's where I see celebrities hanging out, and all the partying and socialization only boosts this illusion I have created, so I would get a slight hint of appreciation, while in reality the only reason I did all of that is so that other people can see the life I'm living, which somehow was supposed to make me happy???

And that very same day, I skipped going to the gym, I had my coffee at home, and went to bed early. The next morning an unusual feeling of relaxation and relief met me as I woke up, and it felt great. Since that day I tried living a more simple, clutter-free life, and I only encountered the concept of the minimalistic lifestyle a couple of months later, on the internet, and after doing some research, I realized something, the chaos I have incorporated in my life, by the presence of unnecessary activities and people only intensified the illusion of happiness, while actually making me feel empty, and that made me try to be like one of those "happy" celebrities even more, but since I started incorporating minimalism in my lifestyle, things changed. All of that chaos calmed down, I trained less, but felt better, I met fewer people, but of higher quality, and somehow I felt happier.

As my day to day life got better, I started reading about this concept of modern minimalism on the internet, and after giving some of them a try, things didn't get much better. I gave up on coffee for a couple of weeks, and it didn't bring me joy, I tried getting rid of plenty of items, only to miss them later... All of those tips and tricks and ideas and opinions are great, but minimalism shouldn't be sold as a blueprint, it is more than a "do that; keep that; trash this; wear that" list, since this lifestyle should be tailored to fit everyone individually, not as a pre-determined ideology.

It's been three years now since I've been living in my own minimalistic way, indeed, some of the ideas mentioned in most minimalism related books and videos are quite effective, but mostly it's my own minimalistic life, not someone else's.

What are you going to learn

First of all, we won't set a straight blueprint for you to follow, in the eyes of the author this is a completely wrong way to get started with minimalism, however, a few commonly accepted ideas will be presented, as their place in the life of any minimalistic living person is reserved.

We'll go through the basic principles, the goals, and most importantly how could your minimalistic life look like, and how much happier it will make you. This is not a rulebook, telling you to get rid of most of your belongings, and many "devout" minimalists will tell you it's wrong, but you can then tell them you're happy, and it's all that matters.

Without further to do, let's start the process of de-cluttering your mind and body, by talking about the essentials, those so called basic principles that indeed contribute significantly towards you goal of making order from the current chaos.

Essentials

In order to clarify the steps, we'll go over them individually as a list, to give you a clearer view or what's it like to be a minimalist "theoretically", but by all means we ask you not to take this information as a rule, as mentioned before, all of these steps and guidelines should be tailored for your well-being, and not for the fanatics that live by strict rules, as they are the greatest at lying to themselves about being happy.

Clearing out your wardrobe

Now this is something no minimalist would leave out in a conversation about their lifestyle, and we have to give them some credit, going over your wardrobe is important, but not if it means going into extremes.

For now, let's look at the basics, you do want to make some room in your closet or dressing, and yes, parting from some items can be difficult, but again, you have options, and don't have to donate them if you don't feel like doing so. Your options are mainly donating or placing the items you consider so in a deposit or box them up and leave them in the attic or basement, but what items should you actually discard?

First of all, go through your wardrobe and scout out the items that no longer fit, those carry a guarantee that you'll never wear them again out of the sheer impossibility.

Next, take a second look through your items, and stop at each one and ask, when did you wear that item last time? If the answer is more than one year, that item should probably get discarded as well. One year indicates that you didn't wear the item in none of the four seasons, and that you probably won't wear it this year either, meaning it's clutter.

Often times people will talk about only having a certain number of clothes, or restricting themselves to a specific palette of colors, mostly white, gray, black and light pastels, which, in our opinion is completely wrong, or more like extreme, since the way we perceive colors, and what they represent to us is a subjective matter, and one should not interpret it in others' light.

By all means, if you are someone who prefers light pastel colors by default, then go ahead and give it a try, but if you resonate with a more colorful look, don't be fooled by the generalized idea of a minimalistic wardrobe, since this is the whole point of "tailored minimalism", to optimize the minimalistic lifestyle so it best fits you.

De-clutter your living space

Another term used and heard maybe too often, is the idea of de-cluttering, by getting rid of all items that you own, which don't "bring you joy". An idea taken to the extreme, in our opinion, as most items, are not meant to "bring joy", but rather to make life easier, and to fit your vision.

Again, you will encounter people claiming that you need to limit yourself to owning only a determined number of items, most often 100, or that those should all fit in a certain window of visual and practical calm, complete nonsense if you ask us.

Indeed, getting rid of some completely useless items is important, such as old papers and assignments that you won't ever need again, or old hardware that hasn't been used in ages, but taking this to the extreme will make you end up frustrating over needing something you just thrashed. One relatively interesting principle in minimalism is the idea of getting rid of duplicates. One we agree with. Let's say you own two identical spatulas, silly example intended, but you will never need to flip pancakes with both hands, so one should go. This applies for anything you own duplicates of but will never have to use both.

Also, take a look around each room you live in, and pay great focus to the decorative items, leaving plants aside. Look at each item individually, and ask yourself, do you really think it looks good, or that it improves the general look of the space, or that the place might look better without it? If unsure, don't thrash the item yet, as other guides might tell you, just set it aside, don't leave it in view for a week, and at the end of it, ask yourself, did you even notice it was missing? If so, you might consider keeping it for a little longer, but if you've forgotten about the item in one week, it should probably be left aside from now on.

Quality over quantity

As a last guideline focused around your surroundings, the idea of giving up plenty of low-quality products and opting for fewer high-quality ones is the only principle we can totally agree with, as it applies for anything, clothes, tools, hardware, furniture and people.

Part of your wardrobe and living space de-cluttering could also be the replacement of some individual pieces with multi-functional ones, the same way a smartphone is now also a camera, calculator, calendar, phone and library, one multi-functional tool can replace a whole set of screwdrivers for example.

Also, don't run from technology, as some may tell you, the simplest example and also pro argument is the Kindle reader. One device can replace hundreds or even thousands of books. Instead of taking up a whole shelf, it fits in a backpack pocket. Some technological advancements bind really well with the minimalist who's willing to try something new.

A small branch of the quality over quantity principle is to go reusable instead of plastic. Without mentioning the ecological benefits, we'll resume to the minimalistic benefits only. By opting for reusable, a straw for example, the amount of space you save up by having a set of 6 reusable straws (for when you might have guests over) instead of having a full set of 100 plastic straws laying around is considerable, also when you think about the fact that those metal reusable straws will last a lifetime, while the single use ones will eventually end, forcing you to buy new ones. Getting one textile bag, instead of having tens of plastic one laying around is another great step, cups, bottles and any product you can buy reusable of, should be on your list.

Quit smoking and drinking

Here is probably the most difficult part in the whole process of inner de-cluttering. Both drinking and smoking are bad for your health in general, and also addictive. The easiest way to go about this is to actually want to. You won't quit either of these because a book told you to, or because you know how bad they are, that's the exact reason why we only recommend one thing, patience. There is no need to tell you WHY to quit these terrible habits, because, as you advance with the minimalist lifestyle, and tailor it for your fitting, the urge to both tobacco and alcohol will come in time. Personally, I kept smoking for quite some time after discovering minimalism, until suddenly, I felt like quitting, and soon enough I did.

Filter social media and entertainment

By all means the most important step in any minimalist's life, getting rid of negative influence. This book is here to teach you how to mold the minimalist concept to your liking, but for this part, we might have some of the solid rules we've previously mentioned.

Social media was the black plague of society, and minimalism it's renaissance. The idolization of celebrities and so-called "influencers" led to the young generations' development in a society filled with standards and trends, unwritten rules and ideologies, all revolving around the same sinful concept, the idea of "plenty".

Plenty of cash, plenty of people, activities, stuff, brands, ideals, and expectations, all because we, as a society, started idolizing certain people we saw on television in the first place, later, with the advancement in the fields of technology, we ported this behavior to the now well spread social media, where fresh generations of easily influenced teens are bombarded daily with the very same ideals and expectations older generations have been through television.

In conclusion, the first step in killing the problem is to kill its roots. Again through the mentality of tailored minimalism, the choice is yours, either to delete your social media apps and accounts, which is an extreme step, or to just filter them?

With all that bad being said, let's not forget how much good technology brought us, and the best way to go about this, in our opinion is to find the sweet-spot, where only good information comes through, while the pop-culture influences are left out.

The way to go about it is simpler than you'd think. The first step is to open a social media app, such as Instagram, and unfollow each and every page that showcases the concept of "lifestyle". This means celebrities, influencers, car-, house-, and fun-related pages, and also those individuals that you personally know, but are trying to copy either of those.

The next step is to repeat this process with all other social media apps you use.

And now, for the other crucial half, entertainment must be tailored to the sweet-spot as well, and the most convenient way to do that, is to actually get rid of cable television. Truth be told television has become an absolute mess, streaming platforms having taken over the consumers, television is not worth it, nor the quality of the shows or the price, instead, streaming platforms such as Netflix, HBO Go, and Youtube, offer a much better experience, free of charge or advantageously priced, and are packed with infinite hours of educational content. This form of entertainment is not only constructive, but the content is shrunk down in a few-minutes long videos, so your time won't be consumed on the virtual platform.

Quit binge eating

As mentioned, this is as long as environmental minimalism goes, because it's all you need. Most of the joy and happiness minimalism brings you doesn't come from the lack of stuff in your home, but from the implementation of good daily habits and the elimination of bad ones, the first one being binge eating.

Munching on lots of snacks continuously during day and night is in direct opposition with the minimalist life, not only does it make you buy more food, and make you gain weight, it can revert progress significantly, through health and image problems, remember, we are not running or hiding from the flaws in our image, but we are fixing them through minimalism.

Binge eating is a problem that affects millions around the world, causing uncontrollable cravings, lowering self-esteem, increasing unnecessary weight gain, and ruining people's confidence.

Binge eating can be difficult to combat, as people affected by it lose control of their appetite, which can be hard gain back, but by the time you close this book, tackling binge eating will be as easy as simply saying it. Covering the science behind weight gain and cravings, the 7 hacks listed in this book will help you overcome any cravings and appetite disorders in the most effective way possible. Information that will change the way you look at binge eating forever, backed up by science and studies.

How to deal with binge eating?

Binge eating has one major consequence that affects people on a daily basis, weight gain, so the best way to tackle this subject, is the same as any other weight gain/loss topic, through nutritional and progressive information.

All body changing programs, or fitness programs as are more commonly known, use one common principle, change is the result of multiple factors. Just image that you are building a pyramid, and the small changes you make to your lifestyle are the bricks. You will never build a pyramid using only one or two bricks, but by using all of the small tips and hacks you know, simultaneously, will get you the desired results.

Before heading into the 7 hacks to overcome binge eating, let's take a look at how weight gain and loss works, along with some ideal perspectives from a nutritional point of view.

Nutrition is key to any weight loss program. Your body is capable of amazing things, just think about how our body grows and develops in the first 18 years of our life. We are born with only a few pounds, yet, we rapidly develop stronger muscles, our bones grow and strengthen, our whole organism adapts to new challenges. In order to achieve this, however, our body requires certain resources. Humans are omnivore, yet we do need certain vitamins and minerals found only in meat, vegetables, fruits, grains, which, in the XXI. century, we can supplement. One thing to remember is, that no supplement can compete with actual healthy food.

The correlation between eating and gaining / losing weight takes place when it comes to our caloric rate. Most people are familiar with the calorie / kilocalorie measurements, the scientific definition is: "A calorie or calory (archaic) is a unit of energy. Various definitions exist but fall into two broad categories. The first, the small calorie (symbol: cal), is defined as the amount of heat energy needed to raise the temperature of one gram of water by one degree Celsius at a pressure of one atmosphere. The second, the large calorie or kilocalorie (symbols: Cal, kcal), also known as the food calorie and similar names, is defined as the heat energy required to raise the temperature of one kilogram (rather than a gram) of water by one degree Celsius. It is equal to 1,000 small calories."

Our bodies require a certain amount of calories daily, in order to live a healthy life. This number varies from person to person, depending on aspects such as sex, height, weight, age. There are many formulas for calculating our needed caloric intake, the simplest and best option would be to go online and search for " calories calculator ", and fill out an online formula. For people who would like to calculate it themselves, we'll recommend the World Health Organization's 1980 equation.

Formula :

Females: Age 3 to 9 years = 22.5 x (Weight in kg) + 499 Age 10 to 17 years = 12.2 x (Weight in kg) + 746 Age 18 to 29 years = 14.7 x (Weight in kg) + 496 Age 30 to 60 years = 8.7 x (Weight in kg) + 829 Age over 60 years = 10.5 x (Weight in kg) + 596

Males: Age 3 to 9 years = 22.7 x (Weight in kg) + 495 Age 10 to 17 years = 17.5 x (Weight in kg) + 651 Age 18 to 29 years = 15.3 x (Weight in kg) + 679 Age 30 to 60 years = 11.6 x (Weight in kg) + 879 Age over 60 years = 13.5 x (Weight in kg) + 487

Let's say you are a 22 year old female. The average American woman over the age of 20 weighs 168.5 pounds and stands at just above 5 feet 3 inches. Based on this information, by introducing this data into an online calorie intake calculator, assuming you have a sedentary lifestyle with little to no exercise, we'll find out that you need 1,789 calories a day, this number will vary based on your lifestyle activity, that's why we recommend using an online calorie calculator to accurately determine how many you actually need.

This number shows how many calories you have to take in, in order to maintain your weight.

The basic principle of weight gain and loss is simple, you eat less calories than you need, you lose weight, you eat more calories than needed, you gain weight.

Notice we said "you lose weight", not fat. Indeed by eating less calories than you need, you will lose fat, but also muscle. This is why usually an exercise program is recommended when we are trying to lose fat, not only it speeds up the process, but it maintains our muscle mass, and help lose as much fat as possible, while losing as little to no muscle. Another thing worth noting is that we use the term "nutrition", not "diet". The reason behind this is that most fit people, consider eating healthy a lifestyle, while a diet is something you do for a determined period of time.

In the following, we will focus on how to apply these rules, in order to lose fat, depending on your determination and expectations. As we said, you can skip exercising and still lose weight, with a significant part of it being fat.

Essentials

You can find how many calories are in every food on the back of the package, or online. Based on that and using a kitchen scale, you can determine how many calories you took in with every meal. There are countless calorie tracking apps to download to your phone, instead of writing down every meal. We suggest using an app as it makes it a lot easier to keep track of your daily and weekly calories.

Before we dive into the actual nutrition plans, depending on how determined you are, first let's take a look at some foods you should automatically avoid if you are looking to lose weight. These foods are high in calories, have little vitamins and minerals, and are best avoided or substituted for their low-calorie, diet-friendly alternatives.

Soda – any type of beverage, with the exception of water, tea, coffee should be avoided. Also we recommend having tea or coffee with no sugar, or, with artificial sweeteners, like Stevia. The substitute for these drinks would be their 0 sugar versions, which are more unhealthy but have little to no calories.

Pasta – go for whole grain pasta or rice noodles.

Pastry – extremely packed with carbohydrates and calories, not fulfilling, pastry should not touch your plate or mouth if you are aiming for a summer body.

Sweets – anything that falls into the category of desserts, candy, or treats, will be considered an enemy. You can find o sugar chocolate and candy in most supermarkets, usually sweetened with Stevia. Also we will cover many delicious treats for you to eat, that will not harm your physique.

Fast food – another pretty obvious category, no burgers, fires, fried chicken, tacos, or anything you can get at a drive-through should be consumed. Most of the food you eat should be made at home, or, if you are eating out, go for a restaurant, not a fast food place.

Deep fried food – Anything fried in a bunch of oil, from fired chicken to French fries. Their healthy alternatives will be food cooked in the oven, with a little bit of olive oil, and sweet potato fires, made in the oven.

White bread – Replace white bread with whole grain or an even better alternative for a slice of bread would be a rice cake.

White rice – Replace with brown rice.

Alcohol – All alcohol should go, in case you want to have a drink with a special occasion, blonde beer, white wine and gin are the least caloric alcoholic drinks.

Just by giving up on these foods, you could lose a few pounds in a relatively short period of time. A former high school friend lost more than 40 pounds over the course of about 5 months just by giving up on soda, sweets, and bread.

Having sorted out foods that will surely stop you from losing weight, here are a few quick snacks to munch on, whenever you get the cravings.

• A handful of nuts (literally as much as you can fit in one hand)

- Protein shakes (in your desired flavor)

- Popcorn (few calories)

- Greek yoghurt with fresh fruits

- Fruits (excluding grapes and pears for their high sugar content)

- Sugar-free candy

- Protein bars

- Oatmeal

- Rice cakes with orange slices

- Dark chocolate (1-2 squares)

Now, let's dive in the 7 hacks to quit binge eating instantly!

Drink more water

Hydrating yourself is probably the simplest yet most effective way to overcome binge eating. A variety of reasons is present behind this claim, firstly the physical aspect, if you drink more water, you eat less. By filling your stomach with water, less room is available for food, and it works every time. If you want to prove it for yourself, before your next meal, drink 500ml of water, and see how much will you eat, compared to the usual.

Studies show that increased water intake can be linked to weight loss and reduced cravings, as one study conducted on 30 adults, showed that by giving them 500ml of water before eating, they consumed 13% less calories than the group that didn't have water.

Athletes consume more water than the average person, for the highly possible benefits on their physique and performance. Other studies show that water intake can be related to boosting your metabolism, which, along with its fulfilling effect, can make up a significant part of your binge eating stopping process.

Clean your stash

It hardly gets more effective than this, because even if you'd want to binge eat, you won't be able to. Getting rid of any junk food that lies around in your house will restrict your unhealthy options and direct you towards a healthier diet.

Your main target should be chips, sweets, bakery products, pre-packaged meats, sugary treats, and anything else that you might binge on. Swapping these products for fruits and vegetables, or even low-calorie alternatives, such as chocolate sweetened with Stevia, or replacing all white flour products with whole grain will drastically restrict your options, so next time you want to binge eat, you will do so on a fruits or veggies, which won't affect your weight.

Get proper sleep

One of the reasons why teenagers and young adults tend to be fat, or should we say more fat than the previous generations is lack of sleep. Sleep is strongly believed by scientists to be linked with the levels of ghrelin and leptin hormones. Lack of sleep increases the levels of ghrelin, the hormone responsible for the feeling of hunger, while also decreasing leptin, the hormone which promotes the sensation of fullness.

The combination of these actions greatly affects any weight loss program or binge eating control, so tonight maybe skip one or two episodes of your favorite Netflix series, and end the group chat earlier, because the recommended sleep duration is 8 hours, in order to control hunger and decrease binge eating.

Studies concluded that sleeping less than 8 hours per night is strongly linked to higher bodyweight.

Increase protein intake

Protein and fiber are both scientifically proven to help with bodyweight and cravings related problems, so let's look at both separately.

Protein is the most precious nutrient for bodybuilders and fitness enthusiasts, and for good reason. It's the main nutrient associated with muscle gain, increased metabolism, and promoting fullness. A study which had their subjects increase their protein intake by 15% not only showed decreased bodyweight and fat mass, but also a reduced daily calorie intake, by an average of 440 calories.

Some common protein rich foods are eggs, tuna, chicken breast, protein shakes and fish, all of them are great for any weight loss program.

Eating more fiber

Fiber moves slowly through your digestive tract, making you feel full for longer. Fiber is just pure magic when it comes to cutting craving, reducing bingeing and calorie intake, as it makes us feel fuller, and for a longer period of time, and countless studies back this up. The best thing about fiber is how inexpensive it is, fruits, vegetables, whole grains, all of them are packed with fiber, but possibly the best option when it comes to this superstar of foods, is oatmeal. Oatmeal is super cheap, and can be prepared in a variety of ways, depending on your personal preference, form protein oats to fruit oats, its completely up to you.

Eat on a schedule

Programming your meals to specific times each day creates a routine, a routine creates a habit, and habits create a lifestyle. Scheduling your meals to exact times during the day and sticking to that plan will subconsciously change the way you look at binge eating, and will greatly remove any cravings that may mess up your meal plan.

It's important not to skip meals, especially breakfast. It's not called "the most important meal of the day" for nothing, as breakfast determines how will you eat for the rest of the day. Having a protein and fiber packed meal for breakfast will not only reduce the risk of cravings during the day, it will also keep you feeling full enough, until your next meal.

Be determined

At the end of the day, the most important element to any change, is to want it. If you don't want to quit binge eating enough, you won't be able to.

Implement a spiritual habit

We as humans are spiritual beings, with a tendency to believe in the impossible, paranormal, and un-rational, simply because life was meant to be lived on different levels. Meditation and hypnosis are the most common methods used by people all around the world to achieve spiritual peace, and regardless of any stereotypes or skepticism, we invite you to discover the gorgeous world of self-hypnosis.

Self-hypnosis has been around for as long as humans have. It occurs in many forms, from meditation to therapy, hypnosis is not related to only one field of knowledge. Acclaimed both scientifically and spiritually, the state of hypnosis is one that opens up the mind to the suggestions it gets from de inductor of the state. (In our case the inductor and subject are one and the same) In order to achieve this state (trance) of both body and mind, we have to induce ourselves a state of physical and psychical relaxation and also gain the trust of the inductor. For that we have the so called "script" or "story", which is a text that contains certain key-phrases meant to induce the state of relaxation. The main goal of inducing hypnosis is to become as suggestible as possible. When our mind reaches the state of maximum suggestability, it accepts and executes the suggestions it is given by the voice that induced this state. Also, hypnosis cannot be used to induce any "crazy" ideas such as committing a crime or doing something completely against your persona. So any ideas of inducing hypnosis that have been inspired from fiction movies will probably remain in those movies.

Please note that hypnosis is a skill we develop and train, some may be successful right away, while others may need some practice, that's why in this book we will cover multiple variations of "scripts" for different types of users. Each step will be covered in detail, in a technique developed by a self-thought user, from the real world, which means everyone can achieve hypnosis through these steps.

With all that being said, there are 5 steps to the process :

1. Preparing the area
2. Accepting the idea of hypnosis
3. Inducing the trance
4. Implanting suggestions
5. Ending the trance

Preparing the area

The first step will consist of preparing the area you will be in while you hypnotize yourself, because for the beginning, not any setting is correct, in fact, very few are. The key factor here is comfort, you **have** to be comfortable in the selected area, otherwise it will be especially difficult for beginners to relax enough to induce the state of needed relaxation. The more advanced you get, the less this step will count.

First of all, make sure you can have the room for about 30 minutes all for yourself, no family members, friends or pets entering the room to disturb you. A recommended time of day is about 15 minutes after waking up, or anytime during the day, probably with the exception of the night or before bed. Trying to get in a state of deep relaxation when you are tired, could easily result in you falling directly asleep before getting to the end of the induction.

After choosing a time and space, put your phone on airplane mode, have a cup of water and slip in some comfortable clothes. Something not to warm yet warm enough so you don't feel cold would be perfect, for example : a tank top and sweatpants. Choose where will you be laying, a couch, your bed, anything comfortable will work, yet for beginners their own bed should feel most appropriate. Once you get more skilled at self-hypnosis, any setting that allows sitting will work, from classrooms to public transport, anything will work once you get comfortable playing with hypnosis.

Accepting the idea of hypnosis

For the second step, you will need to make yourself comfortable with what you are about to do. Really, there is no reason for you to feel uncomfortable, but setting the right tone inside yourself will 100% help. The simplest way you can do that is by repeating your facts through the following phrases, also these are facts you have to convince yourself are real, no one can get hypnotized if they don't want to.

- It's something completely normal

- People have been doing it for thousands of years

- I **will** discover a new world of possibilities to improve my life

- I'm going to be in charge because I'm the one giving the suggestions

- I **want** to be hypnotized

- I **will** enjoy this

After repeating these phrases a couple of times, lay down in your bed or couch, in the most comfortable position you can. Usually I lay on my back with a very thin pillow underneath my head, and also a thin cover over my body. Everybody should attempt laying on their back, with the pillow and cover based on their personal preference and comfort level. Now that we've found your position, we can start inducing the trance.

Inducing the trance

Inducing the trance is the soul of the whole process, without it, there is no hypnosis. The first 2 steps lose their importance in time, but this will always remain the core of the process, regardless of how long it takes to induce the state of relaxation and to open your mind to suggestions, everyone will always need to go through this, before actually hypnotizing themselves.

The method consists of you, telling yourself what to imagine, and focus on imagining it as vividly as possible. Every visual element (setting, actions) should be seen in your mind's eye and every feeling (heat, texture) should be imagined as if you actually feel it. Overall, a strong imagination power will be key in this process, and the more you practice the better you are going to get. Some people may be able to imagine and feel everything on the first try, others may be able to imagine each setting, but won't feel any changes in their sense of touch.

To give you an example :

Imagine yourself holding a large, ripe, juicy lemon. This lemon is so large it nearly looks like an orange. It's color is a strong yellow, so strong from how ripe it is, it nearly goes into a very light orange. You're holding this gigantic lemon in your left hand, barely fitting in your palm... In your right hand you have a sharp, shiny, silver knife. A knife so shiny, it's almost like a mirror. Imagine yourself taking the knife and making a deep slice in the gigantic lemon. As the knife penetrates the lemon's skin, it's juice starts to pour out, so much juice is drips all the way down the knife, you can feel it reaching your hand. You feel the juice drip down your hand, all the way to your elbow, while the lemon in your hand keeps giving out more and more juice...

- At this time you may notice your mouth being full of saliva, or at least an increase in salivation

This example is meant to help you classify yourself into one of the following categories :

Vivid imagination : You saw a gigantic lemon getting sliced, and felt it's juice dripping down your arm. Your mouth filled with saliva and you actually had to swallow somewhere mid- or post-reading. If your imagination was this powerful, you will have no problem inducing yourself into the state of hypnosis.

Clear imagination : You saw everything clearly, but you didn't feel anything dripping down your arm and your saliva production didn't change at all. People in this category usually take a bit more time to get to inducing themselves with the state of hypnosis, but it requires minimal training, all while they can still be hypnotized on the first try, with a bit more patience and a longer script

No imagination : You didn't see or feel anything, you just read the short script and kept reading on. In this case, next time pay more attention to what you are reading, as the script starts with the word *"Imagine"* and that's exactly what you should try to do.

Before getting to the actual scripts, there are a few things to remember :

You should learn or at least memorize a good part of the script you will be using, all texts are easy to remember, and after a few readings and tries will lock down on your memory with ease. (The best solution for start would be recording yourself reading the induction, suggestion and ending of the trance, in a calm, tender tone, and replaying that.)

You will develop an inner voice, if you don't already have one, a voice that is reading your thoughts to you. It should be a calm, confident tone, speaking clearly and fluently, but the most important aspect is for it to be relaxing.

Some words are of high importance, thus will be written in **bold** letters. When you get to these words, your inner voice should accentuate them, as they are essential to the script.

When the writing turns red, it means you have to physically do something. Those actions are "tests" for you to see how deep in trance are you, and will soon become proof of the power of hypnosis.

The actual scripts will be written in *italics,* so everything written in normal letters is outside the script, and will mostly consist in explanations.

The Water script

This is the longest and most detailed of all 3. Its repetitive nature allows even the newest users to get comfortable with the sensation of deep relaxation and the physical tests help convince themselves how real and strong hypnosis really is. All text should be imagined as vividly as possible, all feelings should be imagined as felt, until actually felt.

Lay comfortably in your selected space, close your eyes, let go of any thoughts regarding life, and focus on your inner voice.

As you lay comfortably, let me guide you. I am your inner voice, a manifestation of your own mind, talking to you. We are one and the same, so there is no reason for you not to trust me.

Building trust with your inner voice is more important than some may think. Convincing your sub-conscious that it can trust your inner voice, because it is the manifestation of you conscious, and thus there is no possibility it would try to do any harm, will make it a lot easier to focus and accept its suggestions.

Relax *and let go of any stress,* ***relax*** *your body, starting from your toes,* ***relax*** *every muscle, every cell in your toes,* ***relax*** *every muscle, every fiber in your feet,* ***feel***

*them loosen up, feel them **relax**. This sensation of relaxation moves higher in your body, it goes all the way to your knees, feel your calves **relax**, every muscle, fiber, and cell just loosens up and relaxes. This sensation expands further, all the way to your waist, feel your legs, your thighs, your butt **relax**, feel them **relax** and eliminate all stress in every cell. The sensation grows even further, your abdominal muscles loosen up, your chest with its every fiber and cell **relaxes.** This physical relaxation expands to your upper limbs, fell your shoulders free up, feel your biceps and triceps let go of any stress, every muscle in your palms starts to **relax**, all the way up your fingertips. Now this sensation climbs higher, **feel the muscles in your neck relax,** and even higher, **feel all the muscles in your face relax,** and now,,, go to sleep.*

Don't actually go to sleep, keep listening to your inner voice, your body however should maintain this state of profound relaxation. Understand the word "sleep" as a metaphor for "relax deeply" or "trance".

*Open your eyes, and notice that you are in a **big**, white room. There is no furniture or windows in this big, white room, only a door. The walls, floor, ceiling, are completely white. The atmosphere of this room **relaxes** you deeply. **Breathing** the air of this room **relaxes** you deeply. Breathe in... Breathe out... **Every breath** of air you take fills your lungs with the sensation of relaxation, **every breath** is distributed through your lungs and fills your entire body with the feeling of relaxation, feel your body **getting heavier and sinking** into the bed...*

You notice a red door, 3 steps away from you. This door has a silver, shiny doorknob and is waiting for you to open it. You are about to make the first step. The first step towards the door will relax your body twice as much, the moment your foot touches the floor. As you make the first step, and **as your foot touches the floor***, you feel the relaxation flowing into your foot and up your leg, further expanding in your whole body, making in twice as relaxed. The second step will double the weight of your body, will make your body feel twice as heavy and sink further down in your bed. As you make the second step, the moment* **your foot touches the floor***, your body becomes twice as heavy, you can feel it getting heavier, you feel your body sinking in bed. The last step will turn your body twice as limp. The moment your foot will touch the floor, every muscle, fiber and cell in* *your body will relax entirely, making your body twice as limp as it has ever been. You make the last step and you can feel your limbs becoming numb, you can feel your body going completely limp, you can feel your body relax. As you are about to open the red door, you know that touching the silver, shiny doorknob will make your body and mind open up completely to any of my suggestions.* ***As you touch*** *the doorknob you feel the sensation of opening up pouring through your body, originating from your hand that is touching the doorknob. Opening the door, you notice, that behind it, is* ***a long, circular staircase***.

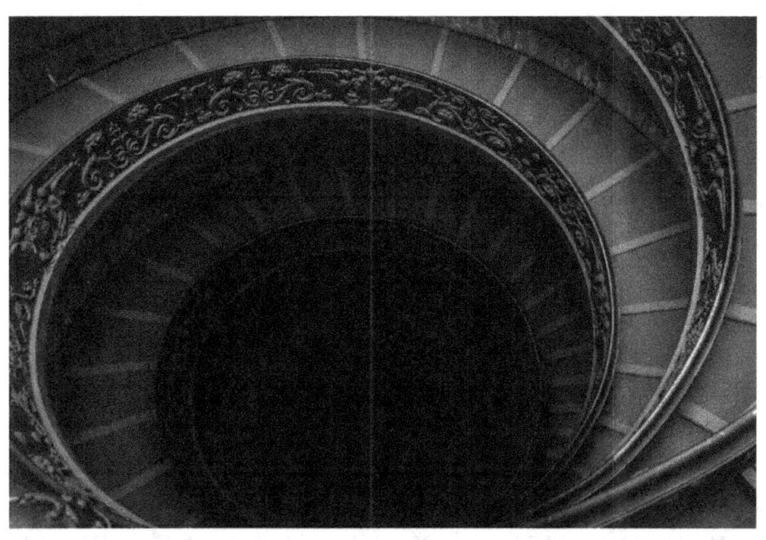

You are standing at the top of the staircase, looking down, you notice that it runs down into complete darkness. Before heading down the staircase, you know that with every step you are going to take, your body will **double its relaxation, weight, and opening to suggestions**. *As you take the first step, you feel your body doubling in relaxation, weight, and opening to suggestions. Now, taking the second step your body becomes again twice as relaxed, twice as heavy, twice as open*

*to suggestions. The third step is taken, your body doubles in relaxation, weight, and opening to suggestions. As you keep heading **downwards**, with each step your body becomes twice as relaxed, twice as heavy, twice as open to suggestions. You keep going down the stairs and you can feel your body get twice as relaxed, twice as heavy, twice as open to suggestions with every step, and every second, it just gets twice as relaxed, twice as heavy, twice as open to suggestions. You can imagine yourself **descending** on this staircase, and as you get deeper down, so does your body get twice as relaxed, twice as heavy, twice as open to suggestions, with each time more and more powerfully. As you reach the middle of the staircase, you stop. In a moment, I will tell you to open your eyes, stick your hands together, and imagine those hands being glued together. As you stick your hands together, you will feel* *them stick together, almost as if glued, and you won't be able to pull them apart. The harder you will try to pull them apart the harder they stick together,* now, as you lay back comfortably, stick your hands together, and imagine them getting glued one to another, with a glue so powerful, nothing can pull it apart. Now take a deep breath in, imagine those hands being glued together, breath out, your hands are glued together with the worlds' strongest glue and nothing can pull them apart. Take a deep breath and open your eyes, as you try to separate your hand you will find it impossible to pull them apart, the harder you try the more impossible it gets, the harder you want to pull them apart the more they stick together. Take a deep breath and go back to sleep. *Your hands are no longer glued together and you can now pull them apart with ease. You will continue to descend the staircase, each step turning your body twice as relaxed, twice as heavy, twice as open to suggestions... You take the next step, and your body becomes twice as relaxed, twice as heavy, twice as open to suggestions... The next step, twice as relaxed, twice as heavy, twice as open to suggestions, and the next step, twice as relaxed, twice as heavy, twice as open to suggestions, you feel your body descend and sink in your bed as well as you feel it become more and more relaxed, heavy and open to suggestions with each step. You keep heading down, your body sinking further into this state of relaxation, heaviness, and suggestion. You keep going down, deeper, taking more and more steps which make your body twice as relaxed, twice as heavy, twice as open to suggestions... Until you reach the end of the stairs. As you reach the end of the staircase you notice a door waiting for you at the end of the last step.*

*You reach to open the door, as you do so, a **warm air** brushes your face from the other side. Opening it you notice that behind the door, is a beach. As you step onto it, the **warm sand** underneath your feet channels relaxation to your body, you feel the relaxation flowing from the sand bellow your feet up your legs, your torso, limbs, neck, and head, relaxing each muscle, fiber, cell in your body. The warm breeze of the beach further relaxes your skin, and overall body. You feel pulled towards the water, so you start walking towards it. With each step you take the sand underneath your feet makes your body twice as relaxed, twice as heavy, twice as open to suggestions, each step, each breath relaxes your body further more. As you get close to the water, your body* *is completely relaxed, and ready for the ultimate state of relaxation. You first step into the water, ankle-deep. As your feet get bellow the water they seem to dissolve, relaxing so much they ultimately vanish. As you step deeper into the water, knee-deep, your calves relax fade away, dissolving in this water. You walk deeper into the water, as it reaches your waist, you notice your lower body has completely dissolved in the relaxation this water offers. The* **warmth** *of this water makes your body fade away from the physical realm... You go deeper into the water, only your neck and head are left out of it. Your torso, shoulders, arms, hands, fingers, all dissolved into the state of liquid relaxation, fading away from the physical realm. In a moment, you will submerge your head underwater. Your neck and head will also dissolve, leaving the physical realm, completely relaxing your mind* *and body. Take a deep breath, and let your head sink underwater. As the water slowly covers your neck, your nose, your forehead, and ultimately your complete body, your head and mind dissolve upon contact with the liquid relaxation. Now, completely underwater, your body has **faded** away, leaving the physical realm, leaving only you and me. Hear my voice, and let me guide you, as we are one and the same..........*

This is the first and longest script, recording yourself reading it slowly in a calm, confident voice is a great alternative to learning it all. After the "........." come the suggestions, we will get to how you should formulate them based on what you desire to accomplish in the next section, for now, let's take a look at the second, shorter script.

The Space script

***Relax** and let go of any stress, **relax** your body, starting from your toes, **relax** every muscle, every cell in your toes, **relax** every muscle, every fiber in your feet, **feel** them loosen up, feel them **relax**. This sensation of relaxation moves higher in your body, it goes all the way to your knees, feel your calves **relax**, every muscle, fiber, and cell just loosens up and relaxes. This sensation expands further, all the way to your waist, feel your legs, your thighs, your butt **relax**, feel them **relax** and eliminate all stress in every cell. The sensation grows even further, your abdominal muscles loosen up, your chest with its every fiber and cell **relaxes.** This physical relaxation expands to your upper limbs, fell your shoulders free up, feel your biceps and triceps let go of any stress, every muscle in your palms starts to **relax**, all the way up your fingertips. Now this sensation climbs higher, **feel the**

muscles in your neck relax, and even higher, **feel all the muscles in your face relax,** and now,,, go to sleep.

Imagine your body as it is now, laying on the most comfortable cushion, deeply relaxed. Your body and mind will leave the earthly realm, see your body slowly lift up, and levitate a few inches off the bed. As your body lifts up, you feel it relax, as if it leaves behind all the stress and tension. Your body will slowly rise higher, and higher. As it ascends, all the tension in your muscles fades away, all the stress gets left behind. Your body rises higher, passing through the ceiling and roof of your house, rising higher and higher, relaxing more and more. Every muscle, fiber and cell in your body relaxes in progressively as your body ascends higher and higher. You see yourself leaving the atmosphere, all *the stress and tension being left behind, and your body feeling completely **limp**. Your body rises higher and higher, and so does the sensation of relaxation. Ultimately your body reaches a stop, and is levitating in the galaxy, **floating**, staying still under a sky covered by stars.*

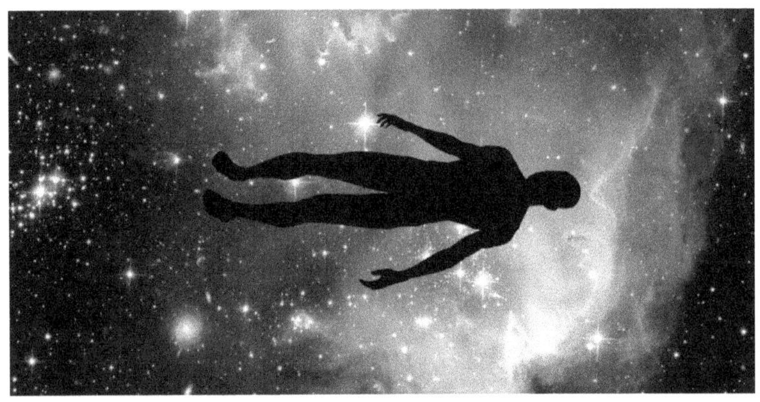

*As your body levitates in the open of the galaxy, the sensation of **relaxation infuses deeply** in every cell of every part of your body. Your body has no mass, it is lighter than a feather, and has opened up to suggestions. As relaxation **flows into it,** you see your body slowly fade*

away... Your body starts getting slightly transparent, further opening to suggestions. The relaxation keeps flowing into your body, fading it away from the physical realm. It is already transparent enough for the stars to shine through it. As your body is barely an outline of its physical form, you open up completely to the power of suggestions, as you see your body **fading completely**, *leaving this realm and becoming one with the* **absolute relaxation.**

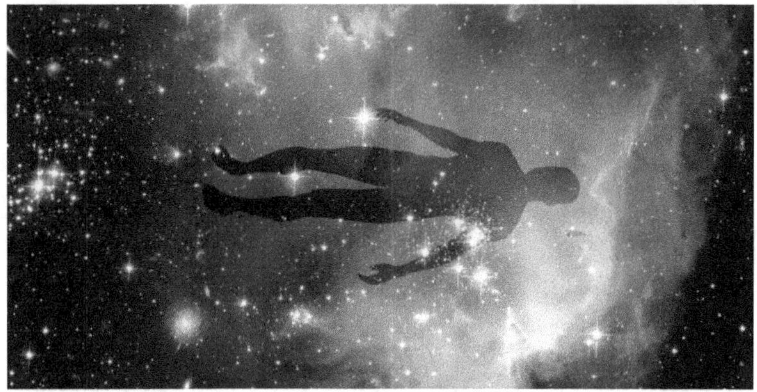

Hear my voice, and let me guide you, as we are one and the same.........

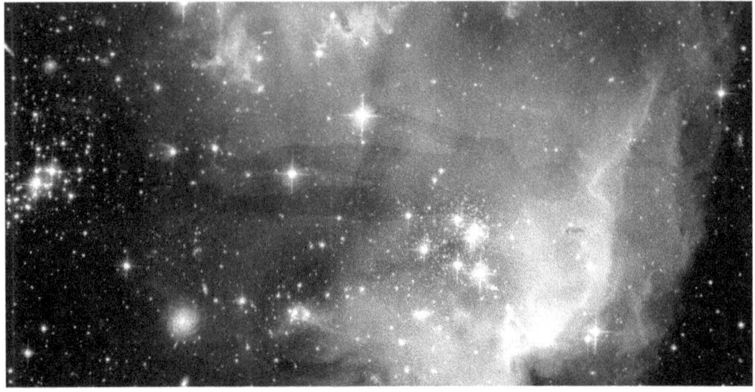

The last thing you should imagine is the human figure fading away completely, the visual representation provided is to help you better imagine the whole setting.

The Power word

A more advanced user of hypnosis can implant themselves with a suggestion, triggered by a specific word. Using this, one can instantly fall into trance, or at least speed up the process, upon hearing the trigger-word. Implanting such a suggestion can take time, and it basically consists of inducing a trance, using whichever script they prefer, and once hypnotized, the only suggestion they give themselves repeatedly is the trigger-word and its effect.

For example : Every time you hear the word " scarlet " , you will...

Some experience with hypnosis is recommended but it differs from person to person. As a personal example, every time I say (out loud or in my inner voice) the word "scarlet", my body goes limp, my muscles relax, and I'm ready to give myself suggestions in less than 2 minutes. The following script is the one I used to implant this trigger-word and its effect. You can use any word you desire, preferably not a very common one.

Relax *and let go of any stress,* **relax** *your body, starting from your toes,* **relax** *every muscle, every cell in your toes,* **relax** *every muscle, every fiber in your feet,* ***feel*** *them loosen up, feel them* **relax**. *This sensation of relaxation moves higher in your body, it goes all the way to your knees, feel your calves* **relax***, every muscle, fiber, and cell just loosens up and relaxes. This sensation expands further, all the way to your waist, feel your legs, your thighs, your butt* **relax***, feel them* **relax** *and eliminate all stress in every cell. The sensation grows even further, your abdominal muscles loosen up, your chest with its every fiber and cell* **relaxes.** *This physical relaxation expands to your upper limbs, fell your shoulders free up, feel your biceps and triceps let go of any stress, every muscle in your palms starts to* **relax***, all the way up your fingertips. Now this sensation climbs higher,* ***feel the***

muscles in your neck relax, and even higher, **feel all the muscles in your face relax,** and now,,, go to sleep.

After using whichever script you find works best for you, Water or Space

      Hear my voice, and let me guide you, as we are one and the same... (your name) , **every time** *you will hear the word (* **your chosen word** *), you will be transported back to this state of absolute relaxation. Upon hearing the word (* **your chosen word** *), every muscle, fiber and cell in your body will relax, your body will feel heavy, your chin will drop onto your chest, you will go to sleep, and your body and mid will open to suggestions. Every time the word (* **your chosen word** *) is heard, you will feel your body relax, from toes to head, it will increase in mass infinitely and will open up instantly for suggestions. The* word **(your chosen word)**, will automatically send you to absolute relaxation, transporting you to trance, opening yourself to any suggestion of mine. From this moment the word **(your chosen word)** will be your trigger word, and it will trigger the trance, absolute relaxation, and peace into your mind and body. Upon hearing the word **(your chosen word)**, every muscle, fiber and cell in your body will relax, your body will feel heavy, your chin will drop onto your chest, you will go to sleep, and your body and mid will open to suggestions. Every time the word **(your chosen word)** is heard, you will feel your body relax, from toes to head, it will increase in mass infinitely and will open up instantly for suggestions. The word **(your chosen word)**, will automatically send you to absolute relaxation, transporting you to trance, opening yourself to any suggestion of *mine. From this moment the word (* **your chosen word** *) will be your trigger word, and it will trigger the trance, absolute relaxation, and peace into your mind and body.*

The repetitive nature of this script is essential in order to successfully implant a thought long-term.

Implanting suggestions

Next, let's take a look at suggestions, for different situations. There are limitless suggestions you can use, based on your needs or desires, the following will be an example to help you understand the structure of a suggestion.

How to construct a suggestion?

There is no determined formula for suggestions, however there are a few structural elements that can make it easier to understand.

Action - Trigger – Reason

These 3 elements are present in nearly every suggestion I give myself, their order may vary, but their presence does not. Let's look at each of them in a bit more detail.

Action : This is the core of the suggestion itself. It's usually a verb, such as "do, do not, will, will not" followed by another verb related to the cause you are looking to fix or improve. An example : *"You will be very productive"*

Trigger : A specific setting, action, situation or word, which starts the action. Triggers can be instant "From this moment" or long term *"When you wake up in the morning"* . They can also be more action-based rather than time-based. *"When your feet touch the floor in the morning"*

Reason : A motive to remind you why are you hypnotizing yourself and with what goal. *"In order to get much better grades"*

Suggestions should have an exaggerated feel to them, repeating the same thing over and over again, maybe using different words or placing the words in different order. To give you an example of a complete suggestion we will use the case above, studying better.

When you wake up *in the morning, and when your* **feet touch the floor**, *your* **productivity** *levels will rocket. The moment your* **feet touch the floor** *you* **will be more productive** *than ever, finishing all assignments, remembering everything you study, your* **productivity will be at its**

***highest.** **In order to get the best grades**, tomorrow, the moment your **feet touch the floor**, you will gain the biggest **boost in productivity** ever, you will study like never before. (Your name) breathe in, tomorrow **when you wake up and your feet touch the floor**, you **will be the most productive** you have ever been, **so you can get the best grades**, exhale.*

Based on this example you can construct suggestions for anything you need, pain relief, anxiety, stress, energy, etc.

Ending the trance

Every session must end somehow, and for that we have 2 scenarios. First, if you are hypnotizing yourself before sleep, just go to sleep. Based on the example above *"you will be the most productive you have ever been, so you can get the best grades, exhale... now go to sleep"*. That simple. You will soon fall asleep, assuming you are in a state of deep relaxation, that won't be a problem.

The other scenario, when you have to get up and keep functioning, requires an ending script. Based on the 3 scripts included in this book, there are only 2 endings, as the last induction does not require one. Advanced users can induce a trans within minutes using their power word, implant a suggestion, and open their eyes, ending the trance just as easily.

Water script

After you've done your suggestion(s) and are ready to get up, this is what your inner voice will be telling you.

Now that you've improved your life with the

suggestion(s), it's time to go back to your physical body, emerge from the water, walking towards the shore. As the water no longer covers your body, the areas above water reappear, as you reach the shore, your whole body materialized back. You start walking back towards the door you got here through, with each step your body becomes more and more solid. Entering the door, you start climbing the stairs, with each step your body becomes more real, more solid, the sensation of absolute relaxation slowly fades off. As you reach the top of the staircase and enter the red door, you find yourself in the white room you woke up in. In a moment, you will close your eyes, when I tell you to open them, you will wake up in your room, in the physical world. Breathe in, in a moment I will tell you to open your eyes and you will wake up, no longer susceptible to suggestions, you will no longer be hypnotized, breathe out. Breathe in, you are no longer hypnotized, and it's time to wake up, *open your eyes.*

Space script

Now that you've improved your life with the suggestion(s), it's time to go back to your physical body. Your body materializes back to its physical form, you can see it slowly fade back into existence. With each breath your body becomes more visible, as now the sensation of absolute relaxation fades away. Your body is more and more visible, until it materializes back completely. Now that you've regained your body, it slowly descends back in the room it left. As your body descends the feel of the physical world becomes more vivid, you've already entered the atmosphere, your body feels like before we started. Your body floats back to the room, passing through the ceiling and roof, descending back on the spot it left.

As you lay comfortably, you notice that you are no longer hypnotized. In a moment, you will close your eyes, when I tell you to open them, you will wake up in your room, in the physical world. Breathe in, in a moment I will tell you to open your eyes and you will wake up, no longer susceptible to suggestions, you will no longer be hypnotized, breathe out. Breathe in, you are no longer hypnotized, and it's time to wake up, open your eyes.

You've just made your first steps in the world of hypnosis, a world which as soon as you successfully start to discover, you'll never want to live without. Practice constantly, play around with different suggestions, different scripts, and sooner than you might think you will unlock a shortcut to achieve happiness, while being in conformity with the minimalist lifestyle you're living.

Tailor Minimalism

The whole summary of this books lies in these final pages. We hope you've got a better understanding of how minimalism should be approached, it's a lifestyle, not a blueprint, adapt each idea and principle other minimalists may tell you about to fit you, and you only.

The best method to do this is the 2 week check, which consists of mostly trying out different ideas, and living with them for 2 weeks. After this trial period, ask yourself, "Did it make me happier? Or did it make me less happy?"

Most people fail with minimalism because they adapt each idea and tip they get right away, and end up in the wake of missing their items, missing their friends, missing their life, and ultimately missing their happiness.

Adapting minimalism is a major change, and should be make in baby-steps, that's why both a physical and spiritual change are required, and we advise all readers, who feel ready to implement these practices in their life, to take it slowly, and be patient, only you can know when you're happy, and only you can tailor this lifestyle to best fit you.